Hand sanitizer gel

And other simple recipes for personal and home care based on essential oils

Cosetta Poli

ISBN: 9798635580530

Premise

The recipes presented in this book base their effectiveness on the antibacterial, antiseptic, antiviral properties of the natural essential oils of some botanical species.

Other ingredients contained in the proposed preparations, when not specified, are intended exclusively as carriers, useful for dissolving and transporting the active ingredients homogeneously throughout the preparation.

For example, the alcoholic part contained in some of the suggested recipes, is not used for its disinfectant properties but as a solvent for oils which otherwise could not be homogeneously dispersed in water or gel extracted from plants.

I have selected a few safe essential oils for the recipes suggested usually considered well tolerated and without toxic effects, obviously it is necessary to respect the recommended dosages.

Notice that even essential oils, despite their natural characteristics, can cause allergic reactions. Before using them diluted in personal care products, take care to do a small test.

Essential oils should be handled with care, kept away from children and pets.

4

If you wish to test these recipes changing the suggested essence with another of your liking, find out about the medicinal properties, the dilutions and the possible toxicity of the essence in question.

N.B: products based on essential oils are not appropriate for use on children under the age of 4.

Table of Contents

Reasons to prepare disinfectants and detergents at home

On the shelves of our supermarkets we can find specific chemical products formulated for every situation, for washing, cleaning and disinfecting.

Advertising teaches us that we need everything and nobody pushes us to use few products capable of solving multiple needs and wants.

Essential oils can help us if properly selected for their antiseptic, disinfectant, antiviral, antibiotic properties. Even with a single small bottle of 10ml essential oil, we can easily produce a large quantity of detergent and sanitizing solutions appropriate for home and personal care.

In the recipes included in this book, I have chosen to use only a few easily available ingredients.

Essential oils have been selected for their effectiveness, easy availability and low cost.

The price of the essences is roughly determined

by the availability of the plants that make up the raw material, by their yield (quantity of oil obtained compared to the weight of the herbs), by the costs of the extraction process, of the packaging and distribution.

You can buy them in herbal stores, pharmacies or natural food stores.

As you browse the internet, rely on well-known brands, tested, with a good reputation. Always check the labels.

Packaging must be in dark or blue glass. Pure essential oils can actually damage the plastic of which they are solvents, and therefore become contaminated.

This risk is considerably reduced when we use them extremely diluted as in our preparations, but it is still preferable, when possible, to use glass containers also for creams, oils and sprays that contain them.

A contribution to the environment

Even though essential oils are highly concentrated products and therefore potentially polluting or toxic in case of inappropriate use, they have limitless advantages.

They are natural and biodegradable products, and the quantities needed to prepare liters of product are really small.

By replacing them with detergents you will have a healthier and less dirty home on surfaces and in the air.

You will dispose fewer chemicals in household drains with assured environmental benefits.

The exhalations produced during use are reduced to a pleasant natural perfume, sometimes balsamic or curative, both for the body and for the mind.

Preparing in this way our disinfectant detergents will allow us to eliminate large quantities of plastic packaging from our purchases.

Less disposable bottles at home, more order, more space, less waste to manage.

The advantage is personal, for the community and for the planet.

Does natural cleaning cost more?

A more natural style in the approach to body and home hygiene will save you money.

Even if at first glance some of the proposed ingredients may seem more expensive than ordinary supermarket chemical disinfectants and detergents, their yield is not comparable.

Take for example a 10 ml bottle of pure lemon essential oil:

I can find online a bio product starting from 5 Euros.

Calculating that 1 ml of liquid contains on average 20 drops, we will have about 200 drops of essence.

A recipe that includes the use of 8 drops of essence can be repeated 25 times at a cost of 20

cents. The price can be further reduced by purchasing larger essence packs.

Baking soda: price starting from 80 cents per 500

gr. (0.016 cents per gram)

Marseille soap: net price per 100 grams starting from 0.93 cents with Vegan certified quality.

Perhaps the most expensive ingredient at first glance may be pure alcohol at 90 degrees.The cheapest I have found is priced at 11 Euros for 70 cl.
In our recipes we often use the quantity of a cooking spoon, that is about 15 ml. The bottle will therefore be useful for 46 preparations, at a cost of 0.23 cents per preparation.

Therefore, natural cleaning is effective and do not cost more but it actually save us money. It is all about choosing, no excuses.

Things to check when buying an essential oil

First of all, do not confuse true natural essential oils with chemical fragrances, fragrances that replicate the aroma of plants, flowers and fruits.

Always buy products that have the wording 100% essential oil on the label, the botanical name of the vegetable, the wording "steam distilled" or "cold pressed".

This is the only way to obtain a raw substance that keeps all the peculiarities of the essential oil you wish.

It is always recommended to use pure and not previously diluted products, for example for cosmetic use, to have a better control of the dosage, for an assured efficacy and to not make cleaning operations difficult by dirtying with non-volatile carrier oil the surfaces that we would like to clean instead.

Pure essential oils are extremely evanescent products. To avoid quick evaporation and to transfer the therapeutic and sanitizing properties in every part of the product and in the right dose we need to convey them through other substances, in which they are soluble and that keep them fresh, active and available for our needs.

Essential oils and their properties

Lemon (Citrus Limonium)

It is an essential oil obtained from the pressing of the peel of the fruits with a fresh and sparkling perfume that can help us in many situations, suitable for sanitizing the whole house, but great for the kitchen where it neutralize the most persistent odors of food or fried.

We use it in our recipes for its proven <u>bactericidal and antiseptic</u> properties.

The disinfectant preparations have other qualities too: we use them to sanitize the kitchen or the floors and to eliminate ants and other insects.

 Using the lemon cleanser in work or study environments we will have a natural support for mental work.

Disinfecting the hands with the lemon gel will gradually bleach them and the nails will be strengthened.

Lemon essential oil has qualities that make it an excellent resource in everyday life.

Try these simple tips:

To have a perfumed laundry and a sanitized washing machine, put a few drops of lemon essential oil in the softener compartment.

Dishwasher: to have bright dishes and to disinfect and eliminate unpleasant odors, replace the rinse aid with alcohol vinegar and add 2/3 drops of lemon essential oil.

Removing old labels from glass jars: Immerse in hot water with a few drops of essence, or spread the label with coconut oil previously mixed with lemon oil.

For personal care:

For the treatment of oily skin, you can take advantage of its purifying qualities by adding a few drops to the face cleanser.

A few drops in the shampoo help keeping greasy

<u>hair</u> light and shiny.

Lavender (Lavandula Officinalis)

The smell of clean that reminds us the freshness of freshly made laundry and the cabinets of the past.

The lavender essential oil, obtained by steam distillation, is used in our recipes for its <u>antiseptic</u> and <u>bactericidal</u> properties.

In addition to being able to disinfect, cleaning your rooms with preparations that contain this essence, you will get a comfortable environment, especially in the bedroom, where you can benefit from its relaxing properties and promote good sleep, naturally counteract stress and anxiety, relieve migraines.

By using your preparations to sanitize and refresh the wardrobe (also for men) you will also have a mothproof effect. The fresh and dry scent of lavender is unisex and commonly used in perfumery.

The essence, if inserted in the hand sanitizer gel,

heals any sores, cuts and small burns.

Other uses of lavender essence:

Lavender oil is an excellent <u>mothproof</u>, just pour a few drops on a cotton ball or a tissue to be inserted between the sweaters or in the pockets of the woolen clothes.

In case of <u>ink stains</u> on fabrics try to remove them by moistening the fabric with essential oil, just rub and the ink will dissolve, then wash the fabric as usual. Repeat the operation if necessary.

Tea Tree (Malaleuca Alternifolia)

<u>Antibacterial, antifungal, antiseptic, antiviral.</u> These are the properties that make tea tree essential oil perfect for your preparations.

The essence obtained from this Australian plant is now well known and searched for its important properties, for the few contraindications and ease of use. It is one of the very few essences that can also be used pure to disinfect the skin, as it is normally well tolerated.

Very effective, it has a pungent smell that not everyone loves. When your preparations contain this essence, they are ideal for cleaning the bathroom and are effective in environments where mold develops, which are easily eliminated along with their smell.

If the properties of the tea tree are right for you but you do not like the smell, consider creating a mix of essences to make it more pleasant, you could try it with lemon for example. The total number of essence drops to be used remains unchanged.

As an ingredient in the recipe for hand sanitizer, tea tree treats nicks, insect bites, boils and helps in case of mycosis.

A small amount of pure essence is an excellent topical remedy in case of cold sores, to be used at the first symptoms only on the affected part by touching it with a muffled stick.

Citronella (Cymbopogon nardus)

Popular for its property of keeping mosquitoes away, we find it easily on the market in the form of outdoor candles or as part of various insect repellents.

However, citronella also has antiseptic and antifungal properties, that's why we can use it as an ingredient in our recipes.

If you use it to prepare household cleaners, in addition to the fresh clean scent, you can benefit from its relaxing properties.

The plant is traditionally used in the countries of origin for the treatment of colds and flu. In aromatherapy it is considered relaxing and useful in case of headache.

Citronella is traditionally used mixed with lavender to create the authentic fragrance of the famous "Marseille soap", if you love this ancient aroma and the sensation of clean freshness that accompanies it, use this information to create your mix for the home.

Eucalyptus (eucalyptus radiata)

Eucalyptus is a well-known plant used for its balsamic effects. The essence lends itself as an ingredient in many industrial preparations, from candies to cough ointments or mouthwashes.

 It has <u>mucolytic, expectorant, anti-inflammatory and antiviral</u> properties active in the specific field of colds that affect bronchi and lungs.

<u>Antibacterial and immunostimulant</u>, eucalyptus is a precious ingredient for personal and home hygiene.

Its fresh scent besides sanitizing all surfaces will make the air balsamic and healthy.

Using preparations containing eucalyptus will protect your pets and your home from insects and parasites.

Other ingredients in the recipes

Food grade ethyl alcohol:

Alcohol from liquors at 90°, commonly called in Italy "buon gusto" (good taste). Is alcohol sold for the home preparation of alcoholic beverages, available in supermarkets and grocery stores.

We will use it in some disinfectant recipes for external use, for its purity and because it does not leave coloring residues, unpleasant odors, toxic residues that we would find in denatured alcohol.

Denatured alcohol:

It is pink alcohol that we normally find in the detergent department of any supermarket. It is alcohol not for human consumption as it is mixed with chemicals and dyes used to make it easily recognizable. Denaturation is carried out exclusively to allow its sale with lower taxation compared with alcohol for liquors.

In our recipes we will use it in minimal quantities, as an oil solvent, only for preparations used for cleaning floors and large surfaces.

Aloe vera gel:

Is a natural gel with countless properties, easy to find on sale as a fresh food supplement oras a stabilized gel for cosmetic use.
It has calming, moisturizing, anti-inflammatory and regenerating properties that will be precious in the preparation of the hand sanitizer gel, which will be rich in cosmetic properties.

If you choose to use food-grade gel as an ingredient, remember that it is a perishable product, which once opened must be kept in the refrigerator.

The recipes include other ingredients that will improve their conservation but I still recommend you to prepare it often and in small quantities.

On the other hand, if you choose the gel for cosmetic use, be careful to read the label, buy a product without fragrance.

Check and respect the expiration date once the container has been opened.

Baking soda:

Baking soda is itself a very useful ingredient for home and personal care.

It deodorizes, cleans, bleaches, eliminates limestone in your home and also has antibacterial properties. It is extremely versatile so it can be used in countless ways, from sanitizing shoes to cleaning the refrigerator.

For body hygiene it is used on skin and hair, for cleaning teeth, in bath water, for foot baths. It is water soluble and economic.

All these properties make it precious to use also in our preparations.

Vinegar:

The acetic acid contained in the cooking vinegar is an excellent disinfectant resource for your home; it is also a splendid degreasing resource, especially useful in the kitchen and bathroom where it will help us by counteracting the formation of limestone.

Not everyone loves its pungent smell but actually, in combination with essential oils, it is possible to use it in minimal quantities and can replace alcohol in recipes if necessary (it does not completely dissolve the essences, but they are sufficiently dispersed).

The best vinegar for cleaning is alcohol vinegar, colorless and strong, but if you prefer a more delicate vinegar and a less aggressive product, apple cider vinegar can be a valid substitute.

Coconut oil:

Coconut edible oil is a precious carrier oil, perfect for welcoming and enhancing the characteristics of essential oils. It has antifungal, antiviral and antibacterial properties. It does not go rancid, and below 25 degrees it has a compact and buttery consistency. It can be warm, and once liquefied it is ready to perfectly welcome and dilute the essences.

Coconut oil has numerous applications in the cosmetic field, for skin and hair.

Its characteristics make it an active ingredient

and perfect diluent at the same time, ideal in the cretion of your hand disinfectant cream, which will have nourishing and emollient properties.

In the cold season it can be safely used in wide-mouth jars, with screw closure. It will remain solid and will not tip over if carried in a bag.

Glycerol:

Glycerol, or vegetable glycerin, is a cheap, versatile and easy to find product, it is used both in the food and cosmetic fields.

Common ingredient in conditioners, creams and masks for hair and skin, it is emollient and moisturizing. It can also be used on skin disorders (eczema, psoriasis, etc.).

In our recipes we also use it for its stabilizing and preserving properties. It is also useful to know that, if necessary, it can replace alcohol in some preparations.

Gel and spray to disinfect hands - 4 recipes

1 - Aloe vera based disinfectant gel (doses per 100ml/0,11qt)

What do you need:

A container, possibly in dark glass (100 ml.) with a dispenser or alternatively a plastic container with dispenser or spout.

- 100 ml (0,11 qt) of aloe vera gel for cosmetic use

- 24 drops of tea tree essential oil or eucalyptus, alternatively use 15 drops of tea tree and 10 of lavender.

Put ingredients in the container and shake very well so that the essential oil mixes also with the gel.

2 – Food grade aloe vera based disinfectant gel.

Aloe gel for internal use is more liquid than preparations for cosmetic use, and in particular it is a perishable product, to be kept in the refrigerator once the container has been opened.

 If you want to use this ingredient, it is preferable to prepare small quantities of disinfectant and replace it often.

To stabilize it use this recipe:

Instructions for preparing 50 ml (0,05 qt) of hand sanitizer:

Fill three quarters of a 50ml (0,05 qt) container with aloe gel add a teaspoon of glycerol.

Close the container and shake it until the ingredients are mixed. Add 14 drops of essential oil. Close and shake once more.

My favorite mixes:

7 drops of lavender and 7 drops of citronella. Or, alternatively, 7 drops of lemon essential oil and 7 of eucalyptus.

3 - Aloe disinfectant gel - alcoholic

Fill half with aloe gel a 100 ml (0,11 qt) container; add a spoonful of glycerol, 25 drops of essential oil of your choice or a mixture of them.

Add liquor food alcohol in the quantity needed to fill the container.

Shake the bottle until the emulsion is homogeneous.

4. Oily hand disinfectant

Using simple food grade coconut oil we can create a nourishing and protective hand sanitizer, which will appear solid in a cold and liquid environment when the temperature exceeds 25°C.

It will be necessary to keep it in a wide-mouthed jar, preferably with a screw closure, in order to use it as a solid and to prevent it from accidentally spilling when it is liquid.

Preparation:

Warm up the desired amount of coconut oil in bain-marie, once it liquefies turn off the stove and pour the ingredients, one spoon at a time, counting the number of spoonfuls of oil, in the small jar with screw cap.

Add 3 or 4 drops of the chosen essential oil (or a mix of multiple oils) to each tablespoon of coconut oil.

If necessary, just collect a small part of oil with your fingers and rub it on your hands, <u>normally coconut oil is quickly absorbed and leaves no trace</u>, but if necessary remove the excess with a tissue.

Other uses: coconut oil and tea tree

By using tea tree essential oil in this preparation, you will obtain an excellent <u>foot care</u> product, useful in case of mycosis of skin and nails.

Also perfect for use as a <u>hair mask</u>: a teaspoon will be enough to nourish and disinfect the scalp.

Combats the formation of dandruff, regenerates and polishes the hair, prevents split ends.

Use it by leaving the mixture on dry scalp and hair for 20 to 30 minutes, then proceed with shampooing as usual.

By using two drops of 100% tea tree essential oil and a teaspoon of baking soda for each tablespoon of oil, you will obtain a soft, cleaning and whitening toothpaste.

Coconut oil alone or slightly medicated with tea tree is appropriate for the practice of oil pulling (prolonged rinses of the mouth for the health of teeth and gums), it is a natural teeth whitener, helps the regeneration of the gums. It has antifungal properties useful in case of thrush.

5. Spray hand sanitizer

Doses for a pack with 100 ml sprayer.

100ml (0,11 qt) bottle, preferably in dark glass, with sprayer.

50 ml (0,05 qt) of edible alcohol.

15 drops of one of the essential oils already described, or a mix of them.

Water.

Preparation:

Transfer the alcohol to the bottle, add the essential oil which will dissolve completely.

Add enough water to reach 100 ml. That will result in a whitish emulsion.

Spray on hands and rub. The alcoholic smell will quickly disappear.

Soap for hands and body

If you want a natural-scented soap with sanitizing properties you can get an excellent product by adding about 25 drops of an essential oil among those proposed to a container of liquid soap (300 ml/ 0,32 qt) without perfume.

The recommended soaps are classic Marseille

and natural Castile, check the labels.

The lavender and tea tree essences are appropriate for intimate hygiene, so you can prepare a specific soap.

House cleaning

Floors (4 recipes)

To have cleaned and sanitized floors without using chemicals you have many possibilities to choose from.

Choose the sanitizing essential oil you prefer, other ingredients can help you with the cleaning operations, such as salt, vinegar, baking soda, Marseille soap.

Use microfiber rags for floors, which retain the right amount of water, collect dirt well and release it when washed.

They can be sterilized by boiling without spoiling,

so you can avoid the use of harsh chemicals that are risky for health and the environment. The secret for the perfect use of essential oils in household cleaning products is to dilute them in other ingredients that make them soluble in water, in order to avoid that the drops of oil float and that our preparation is at times extremely aggressive and at times ineffective.

Floors - recipe n.1

Ingredients:

A spoonful of denatured alcohol

10 drops of essential oil (lemon, lavender, citronella) half a glass of white vinegar.

Process:

Put the alcohol in a glass and add the drops of essential oil. The oil will completely dilute and can be added to ¾ of a bucket of water by completely dissolving.

Add vinegar: it will make the water less hard, degrease and polish the floor.

Clean as usual, it does not require rinsing.

Floors - recipe n.2

Baking soda is a precious product for cleaning the house in an ecological way and can be used as a floor cleaner, you can make it highly disinfectant with the addition of essential oil.

The doses for a bucket of water are:

- half a glass of baking soda

-8 drops of lemon, lavender or eucalyptus essential oil - hot water

Process:

Add the essential oil to the baking soda and mix it so that it disperses well in the powder.

Pour the mixture into hot water, stir so that the powder dissolves quickly.

Wash floors as usual.

Floors - recipe n.3

A small amount of natural Marseille or Castile soap is a useful ingredient for a highly degreasing floor cleaner.

Ingredients for a bucket of water:

-A spoonful of Marseille or Castile liquid soap, or alternatively a spoonful of saturated solid Marseille soap solution.

-8 drops of lavender or citronella essential oil or a mix of the two essences (4 + 4)

- half a glass of alcohol vinegar or apple cider vinegar.

Process:

Add the essential oil to the soap, pour into the bucket and add hot water and vinegar.

The preparation does not usually leave residues to rinse, in case it happens just decrease the quantity of soap.

Floors - recipe n.4

The fastest and easiest way to prepare a natural disinfectant floor cleaner at home is by using common dishwashing detergent. Of course it is an industrial product, but fortunately we can find in any shop also "green" products with environmentally friendly and biodegradable preparations.

These are highly concentrated degreasing compounds, a few drops will be enough for cleaning ceramic or stone floors, the essential oil will make the solution perfumed, disinfectant, and will limit the formation of foam.

Preparation:

Combine 8 drops of essential oil with about half a teaspoon of dishwashing liquid, dissolve the mixture in a bucket of water.

The water in the bucket must present itself with very little foam, it is not possible to quantify exactly the amount of the dish detergent as different brands offer different concentrations.

Spray sanitizer for environment and fabrics

This is a simple and useful product that improves air quality, regenerates environments that have remained closed for a long time, deodorizes and refreshes fabrics without staining or leaving residues.

I also use it to freshen the closet and to humidify the laundry during ironing (not in the iron tank).

For a 750 ml (0,79 qt) bottle with sprayer you will need:

- - the tip of a teaspoon of baking soda.

- - 25 drops of lavender essence.

- - Demineralized water if possible (or the less hard water you have available).

- - A spoonful of edible alcohol

Process:

Heat a little water in a saucepan and dissolve the baking soda in it.

Let it cool down.

In the meantime, put the alcohol in the bottle, add the essential oils, and shake so that the ingredients mix perfectly.

Add the warm water from the saucepan. A

whitish emulsion will form.

Dilute with more water to fill the bottle and close with the sprayer.

This preparation can be used immediately but is even better after a few days, it keeps well for a long time at room temperature.

Spray for washable surfaces, bathroom and kitchen.

If you want a strong and practical multiuse spray for safe and natural hygiene, which can help you to keep limescale stains under control, this is the right recipe for you.

Doses for a 750 ml (0,79 qt) spray bottle:

250 ml (0,26 qt) of alcohol vinegar

500 ml (0,53 qt) of distilled water.

15 drops of essential oil (10 of lemon, 5 tea tree - malaleuca)

Preparation:

Pour first the vinegar into the bottle followed by the essential oils. Close the bottle and shake it to mix the essences in the vinegar melt. Add the water.

Disinfect and deodorize the refrigerator

Lemon essential oil helps us with the cleaning to be done in the kitchen with its fresh and natural scent and its effectiveness.

To eliminate odors from the refrigerator, simply pour a couple of drops of essential oil into a small bowl containing a few tablespoons of baking soda.

Leave the bowl in a corner of the refrigerator until it is effective.

Do not increase the dosage of the essence, the perfume must be delicate and must not overcome the aroma of good food.

Cleaning the oven

Even for difficult cleaning like that of the oven, baking soda and lemon essence are worth trying.

Here's how to do it:

Wet the walls of the oven with a sponge, then distribute with the same squeezed sponge a mixture of baking soda and lemon oil (15 drops).

Close the oven and rinse it the next day, or at least after a few hours.

<u>Bicarbonate and lemon essence can also be used to sanitize wooden cutting boards and kitchen utensils</u>, just rub them with the mixture and rinse thoroughly.

Glass Surface Cleaner

For a 75 cl (0,79qt) bottle, a degreasing and perfumed glass spray is obtained by mixing:

1/3 bottle of alcohol vinegar

2/3 of water

20 drops of essential oil - lemon or eucalyptus.

Disclaimer

In any way the author can be considered responsible in case of injuries caused by the improper or irresponsible use of the preparations and raw materials listed in this book or of any changes and variations practiced by the reader.